Legal & Disclaimer

The information contained in this book and its contents is not designed to replace or take the place of any form of medical or professional advice; and is not meant to replace the need for independent medical, financial, legal or other professional advice or services, as may be required. The content and information in this book has been provided for educational and entertainment purposes only.

The content and information contained in this book has been compiled from sources deemed reliable, and it is accurate to the best of the Author's knowledge, information and belief. However, the Author cannot guarantee its accuracy and validity and cannot be held liable for any errors and/or omissions. Further, changes are periodically made to this book as and when needed. Where appropriate and/or necessary, you must consult a professional (including but not limited to your doctor, attorney, financial advisor or such other professional advisor) before using any of the suggested remedies, techniques, or information in this book.

Upon using the contents and information contained in this book, you agree to hold harmless the Author from and against any damages, costs, and expenses, including any legal fees potentially resulting from the application of any of the information provided by this book. This disclaimer applies to any loss, damages or injury caused by the use and application, whether directly or indirectly, of any advice or information presented, whether for breach of contract, tort, negligence, personal injury, criminal intent, or under any other cause of action.

You agree to accept all risks of using the information presented inside this book.

You agree that by continuing to read this book, where appropriate and/or necessary, you shall consult a professional (including but not limited to your doctor, attorney, or financial advisor or such other advisor as needed) before using any of the suggested remedies, techniques, or information in this book.

Contents

Introduction

In this book we will look at the benefits of a healthy lifestyle as well as the science behind weight gain and fat storage as you age. Giving you an insight into the science behind these especially in your 50's and understanding how menopause can throw your efforts into disarray. These will hopefully help to provide you with more confidence as you move forward on your weight loss journey. There are so many benefits to living a healthy life and losing weight and that you shouldn't let a little thing like your age stop you from getting the body you have always wanted. Not only will you feel healthier but the confidence you gain from looking your best is invaluable.

We will give you exercises to help keep you fit and help you lose that weight. We will start at the beginning with more basic tasks for beginners and will move up to more advanced practices. We will give you a meal plan to follow through your first four weeks of weight loss as well as a section giving you tips and advice on keeping up your hard work, even after your meal plan runs out. This book will equip you with enough knowledge to chart your own fitness journey and plan your exercises.

The good news is the information presented herein is based on real health facts, as experienced by myself. As you may know, I once had weight issues as I was approaching 50. I only know full well the difficulties for many women to maintain a svelte figure at this age. This book won't make false promises on shortcuts, or quick temporary results. Hopefully, this will be the jumpstart you need to live the rest of your life more healthily.

The road to health and fitness over the age of 50 comes with its own unique set of challenges, but it is by no means impossible. There is apparently a lot of confusion and frustration surrounding this topic, but hopefully, this book will shed some much-needed light on it, and become a guide that you can refer to when you may hit a roadblock or hurdle in your journey to weight loss and fitness.

At any age in your life, you should always consider fitness and your weight goals. Being healthy can be an invaluable asset in your day to day life and overall happiness and confidence. Aging is a part of life with its advantages and disadvantages the same as anything else in our lives. Your body will start to react in different ways. Exercises and eating plans that used to work for you might not work anymore.

Society tells us that we lose value as we age. Especially for women, this can be particularly devastating. But what I did not do was flop over and accept my fate. There are many women in their 50's, 60's and beyond who are disproving the myth that your value ends once you are over the age of 50. They are fit, healthy and making enormous contributions to the world.

Many things hinder us in life from achieving our goals, but the main obstacle is ourselves. Anything is possible if you have the desire, drive, and determination to make it happen. You are the architect of your life, and only you can make the change you want. I hope that you reach all of your fitness goals regardless of what age you are right now.

Health, fitness and working out are things that truly excite me and bring immense joy to my life. I love sharing my passions with others, and writing is my preferred avenue for conveying my knowledge and expertise. Many of the workouts featured in this book are some of my personal favorites. I have also included some of my favorite healthy food recipes as well. Follow me as we take the journey to the personal enhancement and getting the body that we've always dreamed of. After reading this book you will no longer look enviously at women with lifted, toned bums. Instead, you will respect and understand the effort they have put into achieving it because you will have done the same.

Thanks again for buying this book, I hope you will enjoy it!

Chapter 1 - Menopause and the Hormones that Might Get Depleted

Menopause is actually a normal process and condition all women will experience as they age. It actually marks the end of your menstrual cycle. The entire menopausal stage involves several changes during the process. It also serves as the end of your reproductive period. Before, the menopausal stage is one of the future phases of my life that I prefer not to experience. I am dreading the day when I'm already reach this period of my life.

While it's a natural physiological process and is not considered a disorder or disease, I heard that some women experienced several unwanted symptoms during the menopausal transition. Some of the symptoms I heard that these women experience, are irritability, moodiness, difficulty sleeping, hot flashes, and painful sexual intercourse. I'm also worried about the fact that there are also women who developed depression because of it.

However, my worries are finally alleviated when I heard that there are also women who never experienced problematic menopausal symptoms at all. Some of them were even able to maintain their excellent physique, and this is something that I'm trying to achieve, too. I think that a full understanding of what menopause is and what you'll go through during the whole process can ease the symptoms and help you manage them well.

So What is Menopause Really?

Just like what has been mentioned earlier, menopause can be defined as that specific stage in your life when your menstrual cycles permanently cease because your ovarian oocytes deplete naturally as you age. It's one of the unavoidable changes in a woman's life, especially if she already has reached middle age. The average age of women who went through the menopausal stage is 51. However, take note that it actually has a wide starting range. You can even expect it to start in your 40s.

To diagnose the menopausal stage, it has to be done in a retrospective manner. The diagnosis is often conducted after you miss your menstrual period for twelve consecutive months. If that happens, then it's indeed the sign that you have permanently ended your fertility.

What are the Signs and Symptoms?

Among the signs and symptoms of menopause that you'll most likely experience are irregular periods, hot flashes, vaginal dryness, chills, sleeping difficulties, mood disorders, night sweats, dry skin, thinning hair, and the loss of the fullness of your breast. You'll also be at risk of gaining weight mainly because of your slowed metabolism and some hormonal changes and depletion.

Hormonal Depletion during Menopause

Hormonal changes and depletion can happen during your menopausal period. The problem with this is that it might also cause you to gain weight. Some of the hormones that might get depleted during this stage of your life, affecting your ability to lose weight or maintain a healthy one, are the following:

- **Estrogen and Progesterone** – These two are considered as the primary female hormones. They work together in ensuring that your reproductive system functions at its best. Estrogen function by controlling your mood while maintaining your insulin, cortisol, and metabolic hormones. Progesterone on the other hand, has sedating and calming effects and works in maintaining the proper balance in your thyroid hormones and insulin.

  The problem is that these hormones might get depleted during menopause. Your ovaries will stop to produce estrogen while your progesterone will stay the same. The result is insulin sensitivity as well as a higher risk of storing more fats around your abdomen. Certain lifestyle changes can help you fight these negative side effects though.

- **Insulin** – Insulin is also an important hormone as it controls the way your body stores or utilizes fat and glucose. A good supply of insulin can send a signal to your fat cells, muscles, and liver to make use of blood glucose for energy. During the menopausal change, you'll experience a decreased sensitivity to insulin caused by the loss of muscles. This will have an effect on your metabolism but rest assured that certain diet and lifestyle stages can counter this.

- **Thyroid hormones** – These hormones are crucial for your body as these control and regulate all your organs and cells. Your thyroid hormones also control your metabolic rate or the speed through which your body functions. They also have a say on the speed through which your body burns calories. Your thyroid hormones might get depleted during your menopausal stage, though. This might result in a slower metabolic rate, which can also have a drastic impact on your ability to lose weight.

Other hormones that might get depleted during menopause that can also affect your weight are leptin and ghrelin – both of which are essential in controlling your appetite. However, I urge you not to worry too much about the depletion of these hormones. With the healthy changes in your lifestyle that I will explain in this book, you can counter the negative effects of menopause on your overall health and weight. It is even possible for you to maintain your healthy figure and feel confident as you age.

Chapter 2 - Benefits and Keys to a Healthy Lifestyle After 50

A healthy lifestyle is crucial to your survival regardless of what age you are in. However, I think that sticking to a healthy lifestyle is all the more important once pass 50. I am fully aware that reaching in your 50s you will experience a decade of significant change. I am even determined to make those years the best stages of my life. But I can't expect to make that happen if I don't stick to a healthy lifestyle, can I? If you are like me who wants to make your 50s among the best years of your life then you have to start changing your lifestyle for the better.

With a healthy lifestyle in your 50s, you'll get the chance to enjoy numerous benefits – one of which is keeping your weight on track. Note that as you reach that age, weight gain is somewhat inevitable, especially because aging women also experience decreased muscle mass. There is also a great possibility for your resting metabolic rate to go down and for you to accumulate excess fats.

You may also experience hormonal changes that can significantly affect your health. You can avoid those issues, by following a strict and healthy lifestyle. It is the key to enjoying a happy, vibrant, and healthy 50s. Here are some of the key points that I think, are really crucial in developing a healthy lifestyle in your 50s:

Proper Diet

One of the vital elements of a healthy lifestyle after 50 that you should carefully stick to is a proper diet. Note that you need to eat the right foods during this age to ensure that you stay healthy while maintaining an ideal weight. The best eating plan, in this case, is that, which focuses more on fruits, whole grains, veggies, lean meats, and low-fat dairy.

Diet plans during this age also require sufficient amounts of healthy fats, like Omega 3 and 6 as well as minimal intake of sodium. It is okay to snack in between meals but choose low-calorie treats. By sticking to a proper diet, you can minimize your risk of dealing with age-related illnesses while boosting your health and wellness. You also have lower chances of putting on too much weight.

Regular Exercise

Staying active through proper regular exercises for your age is also crucial for controlling weight gain and improving your overall health. Moderate exercises can benefit your heart, bones, and muscles during your 50s. I also found out that physical activities can keep your brain working at its best. I'm sure you are aware of how your memory and cognitive function will decline as you age but rest assured that you can prevent that with regular exercises. In fact, a 30-minute brisk walk done thrice weekly is already good enough for your brain.

Adequate Sleep

Once you hit 50, you will realize that quality sleep tends to be elusive since you will be dealing with several hormonal changes as well as age-related muscle and joint stiffness that might disturb your sleep. The good news is that there's no need for you to get too many hours of sleep during that age. In fact, 6-7 hours every day is usually enough. Just make sure that your sleep does not get below that; otherwise, your health and weight might suffer.

Brain Activities

Sticking to a healthy lifestyle on your 50s is also possible with proper brain activities designed to improve your mental health and strength. Aside from physical exercises, I highly advise training and exercising your brain, too, so you can prevent cognitive decline. You can actually train your brain to be active with certain activities, like online brain games, crossword puzzles, or Sudoku.

You can even make it work by trying to learn a new language. Your goal here is to keep engaging your brain during your 50s so you can retain your good memory and reasoning. The good thing about strengthening the brain and improving your mental health is that it also ensures that you don't put on too much weight.

Proper Detoxification and Cleansing

Your healthy lifestyle won't be complete without proper detoxification and cleansing. The whole detoxification and cleansing process actually gives you the chance to eliminate all excess wastes and toxic substances stored in your body. It cleanses your colon and other parts of your body from toxins. This is necessary as you hit 50 to ensure that you embark on a new start towards better health.

Imagine all the toxins and wastes that your body has accumulated all throughout the years. Now is the time to get rid of them so you can start enjoying its numerous benefits, including a higher level of energy and weight loss.

I will elaborate all the mentioned keys to a healthy lifestyle after 50 individually in the next chapters of this book, so you will get a better guidance on how you can incorporate them into your life.

Chapter 3 - The Importance of Proper Nutrition and Diet After 50

As you age, healthy eating can make a significant and positive influence on your overall health. That's why I am serious about sticking to a healthy diet as early as possible and staying with it into your middle age years. I really want to have a better experience as I age. I want to feel better about myself, my body, the healthy choices I make, and I think I can achieve that through proper nutrition and a healthy diet.

Healthy eating can benefit older women. The way you eat can actually make a huge difference in how healthy and happy you feel as you reach that age. It's also a big help in managing potential weight gain. Note that once you hit 50, you'll start to experience weight gain, especially if you have an unhealthy diet. You'll notice the extra weight accumulating around your abdominal area first then spreading towards your arms and legs. It's possible to control that possible weight gain with a healthy meal plan.

In addition, proper nutrition and a healthy diet are crucial after 50 as you need to ingest more nutrients to support your weakening immune system. With a proper diet in place, you can maintain a strong immune system, and prevent age-related conditions and illnesses. It can help you avoid serious health issues associated with age, like osteoporosis, high blood pressure, and Type 2 diabetes.

To ensure that you enjoy all the mentioned benefits of proper nutrition and healthy diet after 50, here are some tips on developing a nutritious and healthy diet plan that perfectly suits your age:

Know What to Eat

Reaching your 50s requires you to take a closer look at all the foods that you put on your plate. You should make it a point to develop a healthy meal plan by ensuring that it contains the following:

- **Fruits and veggies** – Your age may cause your body to be unable to absorb enough essential vitamins and antioxidants. It's possible to solve that problem by simply ingesting more fruits and veggies. Pick those with bright colors as much as possible, including bright reds, yellows, oranges, and greens. The brightness of their colors indicates that they are indeed rich in essential nutrients and vitamins.

- **Dairy products** – A healthy diet plan for women aged 50 and above also includes plenty of dairy products. Note that at this age, your bone density will also most likely diminish. That said, I highly suggest getting more Vitamin D and calcium. That's possible with an increased consumption of dairy. A wise tip is to consume up to 3 8-oz. glasses of milk every day as it provides you with the recommended amount of calcium that you need daily. Other sources of low-fat and non-fat dairy are cheese and yogurt.

- **Whole grains** – Rich in fiber and B-vitamins, whole grains can also make a vital part of your healthy diet. Some of your options are oatmeal, quinoa, and whole wheat breads. Stay away from white pasta, white bread, and refined carbs. In case you need to consume carbs, pick the brown variety rather than the white.

- **Fish** –It's also advisable to include fish in your diet plan. It is because it is rich in Omega-3 fatty acid, which is essential as you age. Some types of fish that you can safely eat are salmon, tuna, and mackerel. Avoid eating too much fish, though. Note that you only need around two servings of fish every week to enjoy its benefits.

- **Lean protein** – Sources of lean protein should also be included in your diet plan. Note that your age makes you prone to cardiovascular diseases, so you need to avoid high-fat meat as much as possible. Choose lean meats, instead. You can also get lean protein from fish, legumes, poultry, nuts, and beans.

By incorporating the mentioned foods in your daily diet, you can make it as healthy as possible.

Reduce your Intake of Salt

Instead of using salt when preparing your recipes, use spices. Note that salt is unhealthy for you as you age. It is because it can cause your body to retain water, thereby raising your chances of dealing with high blood pressure that will eventually trigger heart failure, strokes, and heart attacks. Increasing your intake of salt also raises your risk of dealing with kidney stones, vascular dementia, and osteoporosis. That said, healthy eating during your 50s should include minimizing your intake of foods rich in salt. You can actually boost the flavor of your recipes by using herbs and spices instead of salt.

Choose Unsaturated Fat

Stay away from foods rich in saturated fats as much as possible, and stick to unsaturated fat. In this case, cook your recipes using olive oil and other healthy oils instead of butter. You should also remove meat that has several layers of solid fat from your diet. Bacon should be eaten occasionally as it's also rich in saturated fat, which is bad for your health and can stimulate weight gain.

Eat Foods Rich in Calcium

Being in your 50s and reaching the menopausal stage might increase your risk of dealing with osteoporosis. I figured that it is mainly because you will lack in estrogen during this age. Also, your body will be at risk of breaking down more bones than building them, further putting you at risk of experiencing bone fractures and osteoporosis. That's the main reason why you need to get a good supply of calcium. Among the best sources of calcium that you should include in your meal plan are spinach, kale, yogurt, fat-free or low-fat milk, broccoli, and sardines.

Stay Hydrated

Aside from ensuring that your meal plans contain all the nutrients that your body needs at age 50, it's also advisable to incorporate water into your daily routines. You need it to stay hydrated. Note that water serves as a vital nutrient designed to reduce your risk of dealing with dehydration. Your goal is to consume at least 64 fluid ounces or 8 glasses of water on a daily basis.

Chapter 4 - Creating a 4-week Eating Plan for Effective Weight Loss

Based on the tips mentioned above, here is a 4-week (28-day) eating plan for effective weight loss specially designed for women over 50s.

Day	Breakfast	Lunch	Dinner	Snacks
1	1 serving of your preferred fruit 1 boiled egg 1 slice of toast ½ glass of milk	A medium serving of lean meat 1 slice bread Tomato and lettuce salad without dressing 1 serving of fruit	1 serving of lean meat 1 slice bread 1 potato 1 yellow or green veggie	½ glass of milk Crackers with American cheese
2	½ cup bran flakes 1 small banana 8-oz. skim milk	2 eggs (scrambled) 1 cup fresh veggies ½ cup tropical fruit 1 tortilla (around 6 inches)	½ cup broccoli 3-oz. pork loin chop 6-oz. baked potato	¼ cup granola 6-oz. non-fat yogurt
3	½ cup oatmeal (cooked) 1 cup plain Greek yogurt ½ cup strawberries	2-oz. canned light tuna 1 slice whole-wheat bread ½ cup celery 1 tsp. mayonnaise	2-oz. grilled chicken breast ½ cup cherry tomatoes 2 cups leafy greens	½ cup cantaloupe with some almonds

4	1 slice toast 2 egg whites ½ cup of your preferred fruit	2 slices whole-wheat bread 1 slice reduced fat cheese ½ cup fresh veggies	1 whole-wheat dinner roll Roasted broccoli	1 cup cottage cheese (low-fat)
5	2 slices of wheat toast 1 and ¼ cup fresh strawberries 1 tbsp. peanut butter	2 eggs (scrambled) ½ cup tropical fruit 2 cups lettuce	Grilled chicken 8-oz. skim milk Soup	8-oz. skim milk
6	½ cup oatmeal 1 small orange 8-oz. soy or skim milk	Roast beef sandwich 1 cup sliced cucumber 2 slices of bread	1 cup boiled potato 1 cup cooked carrots 3-oz. round steak	3 cups popcorn (use canola oil)
7	1 pancake (around 4 inches) 1 cup apricots 2 tsps. light jelly	2 eggs (scrambled) ½ cup fruits 1 tortilla (around 6 inches)	2/3 cup brown rice 3 oz. chicken breast 1 cup sliced tomato	8-oz. skim milk
8	½ cup bran flakes 1 small orange 8-oz. skim milk	1/3 cup rice 2 tacos (each one containing ground beef, lettuce, cheddar cheese, green pepper, tomato, and salsa)	2/3 cup pasta with red sauce and 3 meatballs ½ cup carrots	6-oz. non-fat yogurt

9	2 slices of cinnamon toast 8-oz. skim milk 1 tsp. margarine	Corn bread (around 2 inches) ½ cup beef and bean chili 1 cup celery or carrots	3-oz. fish 2 cups sliced tomato 6-oz. baked potato	2 tbsps. raisins
10	1 slice French toast 2 tbsps. sugar-free syrup 4 pecan halves 8-oz. skim milk	½ cup grilled pepper, mushroom and onion 2/3 cup brown rice ½ cup grilled pineapple	3-oz ground beef patty 1 cup radishes, lettuce, and peppers 1 whole-wheat bun	1 small nectarine
11	1 scrambled egg ½ cup orange juice 1 cup hash browns	Taco salad composed of tomato, lettuce, pepper, corn, and black beans 7 tortilla chips	½ cup sweet potato 3-oz. turkey tender 8-oz. skim milk	1 cup grapes
12	3 hard-boiled eggs 1 banana 1 grapefruit 8-oz. skim milk	2 hard-boiled eggs Vegetable salad 1 toast	2-oz. grilled chicken breast Mixed vegetable quinoa	¼ cup cottage cheese

13	1-2 oatmeal and blueberry pancakes 8-oz. skim milk	Tropical chicken salad High-fiber whole-wheat crackers	½ cup cooked brown rice Baked tilapia or 6-oz. baked potato	3 graham cracker squares
14	1 cup oatmeal with strawberries and bananas 1 slice whole-wheat bread 8-oz. skim milk	Peanut butter and banana sandwich (1-2 slices) 1 cup roasted veggies	5-oz. steak 1 cup steamed broccoli 1 small baked potato	½ cup peaches
15	1 scrambled egg 2 slices lean turkey bacon 1-oz. reduced fat cheese	6-oz. chicken breast ¼ avocado 1 cup bell peppers (sliced)	2 cups vegetable salad 6-oz. pork tenderloin	½ cup banana
16	1 cup porridge ½ cup stewed apricots 8-oz. skim milk	2 cups roasted corn, black bean, and avocado salad 1 cup cherry tomatoes	9-oz. lean or cod fish 15 pieces asparagus spears	Greek yogurt
17	2 slices wheat bread 1 boiled egg 8-oz. soy or skim milk	2 cups vegetable salad 6-oz. flank steak 2 tbsps. oil dressing	9-oz. salmon 1 cup broccoli	1 slice white bread with 1 tbsps. of jelly

18	1 cup oatmeal 2 hard-boiled eggs	1 whole-wheat tortilla 6-oz. chicken breast 1 cup salad	8-oz. turkey breast 1 sweet potato	1 apple
19	1 cup bran flakes ¼ cup raisins 8-oz. skim milk	6-oz. canned tuna 1 slice wheat bread 1 tbsp. light mayo	8-oz. chicken breast 1 cup green beans	½ cup walnuts
20	2 poached eggs 1 toast 1 glass fresh fruit juice	2 cups tinned salmon salad ½ cup tropical fruit	1 cup quinoa 8-oz sirloin steak	1-2 pieces of banana
21	1 cup oatmeal 2 hard-boiled eggs 1 toast	5-oz. lean burger ½ avocado 1 whole-wheat bun	6-oz. pork tenderloin 1 cup broccoli	Mozzarella cheese stick
22	1 serving of your preferred fruit 1 boiled egg 1 small banana	1 medium serving of lean meat 2 cups tomato and lettuce salad without dressing	3-oz. pork loin chop 6-oz. baked potato	8-oz. skim milk
23	1 and ¼ cup fresh strawberries ½ cup oatmeal 8-oz. soy or skim milk	2 eggs (scrambled) ½ cup fruits 1 tortilla (around 6 inches)	3-oz. fish 2 cups sliced tomato 6-oz. baked potato	Greek yogurt

24	2 scrambled eggs on toast Jam and butter 1 glass fresh juice	2 slices cold beef sandwiches 1-2 cups tropical fruits	1 medium serving of roasted beef 1 cup sliced tomato	¼ cup raisins
25	½ cup bran flakes 1 small orange 8-oz. skim milk	2-oz. canned light tuna 1 slice whole-wheat bread ½ cup celery	1 serving of lean meat 1 slice bread 1 potato	Crackers with American cheese
26	2 slices of wheat toast 1 and ¼ cup fresh strawberries 1 scrambled egg	2 cups roasted corn, black bean, and avocado salad 1 cup bell peppers (sliced)	2-oz. grilled chicken breast ½ cup cherry tomatoes	1 small nectarine
27	1 slice French toast 2 tbsps. sugar-free syrup 1 cup hash browns 8-oz. skim milk	2 eggs (scrambled) 2 cups lettuce Your preferred fruit	½ cup cooked brown rice 1 serving of baked tilapia	½ cup cantaloupe
28	1 cup oatmeal with strawberries and bananas 1 slice whole-wheat bread 8-oz. skim milk	Roast beef sandwich 1 cup sliced cucumber 1 slice of whole-wheat bread	5-oz. steak 1 cup steamed broccoli 1 small baked potato	¼ cup granola

This 4-week eating plan takes into full consideration the specific needs of women over 50 and helps them ensure that they keep their body in tip-top shape.

Chapter 5 – The Importance of Proper Exercise

Though turning 50 was one of my most dreaded moments, my new goal is to be committed to start a happier life, with renewed vigor, after I hit 50. I know that looking fabulous at 50 and beyond and maintaining my figure is not going to be handed to me on a silver platter. I knew that it will take a lot time and a lot of hard work, which I was willing to work my butt off for.

Benefits of Exercising for Women Over 50

If you are someone who is already physically active before you reached 50 then good for you because you wouldn't struggle too much. However, if you're not that active before then rest assured that it's not too late to start.

There are actually a lot of benefits associated to exercising over 50. Aside from helping you lose weight and maintaining a fit and fab figure at that age, regular physical activities can also help in taming menopausal symptoms (the ones that I would really like to avoid as much as possible). These include sleep issues, joint paints, and hot flashes, among many others.

Proper exercise at 50 is also essential because it helps you prevent the development of certain diseases associated with age, including heart disease, osteoporosis, and diabetes. It gives you full control over your weight and helps you melt belly fat. Regular physical activity can also greatly enhance your level of energy. It's also the key to maintaining an excellent emotional and mental state.

It prevents the difficulties associated to aging that's often caused by an inactive lifestyle. Just make sure that before you do certain exercises, you consult your doctor first and find out if you're at risk of developing heart disease because of certain factors, like high blood pressure, family history, or high cholesterol level.

Some Exercise Tips to Lose Weight at 50

To ensure that you gain all the benefits out of exercising for women over 50, especially all that is relevant to losing weight or maintaining a healthy weight, I have put together some tips to make the activities more beneficial for you:

1. **Take it easy** – Especially if you're just starting out on exercise routines, I highly suggest taking everything easy. Also, being out of shape might cause you to get discouraged at the beginning of your journey. It would be best to commit to starting out with small and easy to achieve goals. It could be simply walking for several days a week, 20 to 30 minutes each time. Once you get used to the routine, you can slowly incorporate other exercises that are safe for your age.

2. **Go for well-rounded activities** – One way to ensure that you're receiving a well-rounded fitness routine is to ensure that it contains three vital elements, stretching, strength training, and aerobic activities. Stretching needs to be incorporated into your routines because it will help you warm up while building the flexibility of your joints. It also works in minimizing your risk of suffering from too much strain or dealing with an injury.

    Strength training is also crucial in building and retaining muscle density while reducing your risk of experiencing back injury. You can begin with hand weights. Do 8-12 reps, which is enough to strengthen posture and improve your strength.

    It is also advisable to commit to doing 20-minute aerobic exercise sessions for 3-4 times every week. Some of the aerobic exercises that you can safely do are swimming, walking, and jogging.

3. **Add variations** – Instead to sticking to the same routines over and over again, I highly encourage you to change it up every once in a while. While there are exercises designed for seniors, you can still incorporate some strenuous forms of activities if you feel like you're capable of doing them safely. You can even incorporate certain physical activities, like golf, gardening, hiking, and brisk walking with your dog in your routines just to vary them a bit.

4. **Challenge yourself** – Make it a point to challenge yourself, too, especially if you start getting used to your workouts in the sense that they are already

too comfortable for you. It's possible to challenge yourself by increasing the intensity, number of reps or sets, or incorporating a more rigorous activity that will help get your heart pumping.

5. **Listen to your body** – Note that since you are already in your 50, you might experience some limitations in the way you handle exercises. Some of the challenges that you might encounter when exercising are joint problems, back pain, and arthritis. That's why you really have to listen to your body when doing your routines. If you already feel some discomfort and pain then stop the exercise right away. It's also advisable to regularly consult your doctor regarding the best exercises for you.

By following all the mentioned tips, you'll have a higher chance of staying fit and fab at 50 through incorporating the right exercises. The next chapter of this book will focus on providing you with some examples of safe exercises designed to help you lose weight and maintain a healthy one even as you hit the critical age.

Chapter 6 – Exercises for Optimal Weight Loss After 50

Exercises for Beginners

- **Basic Squat** – Doing a basic squat involves standing tall first and ensuring that your feet are hip-distance apart. Your toes, hips, and knees should be facing forward, too. The next thing to do is bend your knees. Your buttocks should then be extended backwards. It's as if you're going to sit into one chair. Your knees should also be behind your toes. Your weight, on the other hand, should be planted on your heels. Rise up and do the same steps again. What's good about this basic squat is that it targets your quads, hamstrings, and glutes.

- **Bird Dog** – This simple exercise is ideal for beginners who are already over 50. It targets the back and core and can be performed through simple steps. What you have to do first is to kneel on all fours in a mat. Reach one of your arms forward. Ensure that you stretch its length. While doing so, draw in your abdominals while extending your opposite leg behind you. Do it for 8 to 12 times. After that, you can switch sides.

- **Reverse Chair Crunch** – You can do this exercise each time you're seated. It works effectively in toning your stomach muscles. What you have to do is to sit upright in your chair. Your hands should be positioned in front of your body. Ensure that your weight centers on the bones used for sitting. Lean back. Ensure that the muscles in your abdomen stay tight when doing so. Stay in that position until you notice that your weight transfers to your tailbone. You can the gradually go back to an upright position. Perform 15 reps but make sure to stop each time your lower back feels strained or fatigued.

Intermediate Exercises

- **Curl-ups** – This exercise is ideal for women over 50 who wish to add some strength to their abdominal muscles. To do this, you will need to lie flat with your back on the ground. Your knees also need to point towards the ceiling. Put your hands at the sides and palms against the floor. Once in that position, lift your shoulders slowly from the floor. Do 15 reps of this intermediate exercise 5 days every week.

- **Pelvic lift and tilt** – Another effective exercise that you can do is the pelvic lift and tilt, which works effectively in strengthening and toning your abdominal muscles. You can do the pelvic lift by lying on the floor first and keeping your knees bent. Raise your pelvic slowly towards the ceiling. Stay in that position for approximately 10 seconds then release yourself down to the ground.

  If you want to do the pelvic tilt then you have to lie on the ground first then bend your knees. Tilt up your pelvis gradually. Curl the lower part of your back to the floor. Stay in that position for a max of 10 seconds. To ensure that you gain the best results out of the mentioned exercises in terms of losing weight, make it a point to do 10-20 reps regularly.

- **Forearm Plank** – This moderate form of exercise that a woman over 50 can safely do is helpful in strengthening the core, shoulders, and upper back, and in improving posture. Start by lying on the floor. Your forearms should be the ones that lay flat on the floor while in this position. Your elbows also need to be in direct alignment below your shoulders.

  With your core engaged, lift your body from the floor. Ensure that your forearms stay planted on the floor while your body stays in a straight and direct line starting from the head down to the feet. Ensure that your abdominals stay engaged during this position. Avoid letting your hips drop or rise, too.

Advanced Exercises

- **Rows** – This exercise is a big help in strengthening your back, helping you stay upright even when you age. It's also beneficial in the sense that it tones your biceps. You can use a simple exercise tube with a medium to heavy resistance for this. To do this, use the exercise tubing. Ensure that it features one handle on an end. Connect the central part of the tubing to the hinge of your door. Alternatively, you can use a sturdy object as a means of wrapping it around.

  Once done, you can stand in a staggered position while facing the door hinge. One of your feet should be planted in front of the other to improve your stability. Hold the tubing's handles then step back. Do so until you straighten your arms and notice some tension felt on the exercise tubing. The next step is pulling back the handles while squeezing together your shoulder blades. Pause then gradually go back to your starting position. Perform 3 sets of this exercise composed of around 12-15 reps.

- **Lateral or front raises** – What's so good about this exercise is that it lets your shoulders receive a double workout. It lets you carry weights on both sides as well as in front, thereby targeting all major deltoid muscles. With this workout, you will feel even more confident about your figure. You'll even feel confident wearing a strapless dress. The first step to doing this exercise is to be in a standing position with your feet planted on the floor shoulder-width apart.

  Get the dumbbells and hold one per hand. Keep your arms straight but ensure that you do not lock them out. Raise the dumbbells out to both sides. Make sure that they are positioned parallel to the ground when doing this. Go to the original position slowly. The next step is to raise the dumbbells again straight in front of you. Do the steps from the side and front movement. To gain effective results, perform around 2-3 sets of this exercise with 10-12 repetitions each.

- **Seated Overhead Press** – You can also include the seated overhead press as a part of your regular workout routines. One major benefit of this exercise is that it works in increasing your lean muscle mass, especially around your shoulders. This is actually a good thing if you want to lessen your risk of dealing with lower back, shoulder, and neck injuries in case you need to press on a heavy object overhead.

Start this exercise in a seated position. Ensure that your back is properly supported. Let dumbbells (around 5 to 8 lbs. each) rest on your shoulders. Sit tall while positioning your elbows under your wrists. The next step is to press upward in the sense that your elbows are not out on the sides but in the front part of your body.

End this position by letting the dumbbells stay over your head directly. Your palms should face forward and your elbows should be extended fully, instead of being locked. Release slowly but make sure to stick to a similar pattern motion. End this with the beginning position to complete one repetition. Your goal should be to complete 10 to 12 repetitions of this exercise.

Doing any of these exercises on a regular basis can help you maintain an excellent figure even after you reach the age of 50. Make it a point to vary your exercises to keep on challenging your muscles and body parts.

Chapter 7 – Challenges Associated to Losing Weight After 50

I know how important it is to maintain a healthy weight when one ages – that's why I am working hard to stick to a healthy lifestyle as much as possible. Note that excess weight coupled with the stress and pressures associated with aging can cause one to be more prone to developing certain illnesses. It might also shorten one's life. With that in mind, I encourage you to let go of poor lifestyle habits as early as possible.

However, note that once you hit 50, losing the excess weight will be a bit harder. It's not as easy during your 20s and 30s, which just involves doing some minor changes to your level of activity and eating habits. Weight loss during this stage requires more hard work and effort because you might encounter the following challenges:

Aging Muscles

As you age, your muscle tissues also have the tendency of shrinking naturally and losing their mass. While the specific reason for this challenge is still unknown, I noticed that it's mainly because of the muscles' wear and tear as well as the hormonal changes a woman encounters while she ages. The combination of these problems makes your body less efficient when it comes to replenishing any damaged or injured muscle cells.

The problem with your diminished muscle cells is that it can cause unburned calories to convert to fats. In this case, you may have a hard time losing weight because your tendons, ligaments, and muscles also become rigid as you age. They also have the tendency of losing their tone.

Physical Strain

Aging might also cause you to have a difficult time losing weight because you may encounter physical strain. This might cause a decline in your regular physical activities. It is greatly possible for you to no longer be able to perform those activities that you once loved and enjoyed. One example is that running may become strenuous for you, so you might need to trade it with walking. You might also need to replace weight lifting with yoga.

In this case, you may need to perform low-impact activities. This is a bit challenging because this might require you to do the workouts for a longer period or more, pretty often so you can attain similar results.

Hormonal Changes

Another challenge that you might encounter when losing weight at 50 is the hormonal change. While hormonal changes linked to menopause among women do not necessarily cause you to gain weight in an instant, they still have the tendency of causing some changes on the specific areas where you store fats. This results in the accumulation of excess weight in your abdomen instead of other parts of your body, like your thighs or hips.

Hormonal changes might also affect your emotions, which might cause you to make poor choices in terms of diet and physical activities. These changes also have the tendency of triggering muscle loss, which can lead to slow metabolism and reduced movement.

Still, with proper commitment to the right diet and regular exercise, I am pretty sure that all the weight loss challenges after 50 can be easily dealt with. The key to handling these challenges is awareness. You have to be aware of these weight loss challenges, acknowledge that they indeed exist, and figure out how to deal with them the right way.

Chapter 8 – Habits that will Drain your Fountain of Youth

Aside from learning about the specific weight loss challenges that you might encounter at 50, I also highly advise you to gain a full understanding about the different habits that have had in the past which can really sap your fountain of youth. Here are 5 unhealthy habits that might cause you to age even faster. Avoid them as much as possible and increase your chance of aging beautifully.

Crash Dieting

Everyone loves the idea of losing weight in an instant. Who does not want to lose up to 10 lbs. in time for a special occasion? Quick weight loss fixes are very tempting. However, remember that a crash diet is not a great idea. It won't solve your problem for the long-term.

What it does, instead, is that it causes a long-term threat. It even has the tendency of making you feel older because it reduces the level of your energy, causes irritation and depression, and messes your focus and concentration. A crash diet also causes your skin to sag even more and develop more wrinkles. It is mainly because your less elastic skin caused by your age may not have enough time to adjust to the lost weight.

While managing your weight is crucial, especially once pass 50, it's still necessary to go the safe and slow route. Avoid losing over 1-2 lbs. every week.

Inadequate Sleep

Another habit that you should avoid if you want to age gracefully is not getting the right amount of sleep. Note that inadequate sleep can prevent you from functioning optimally all throughout the day. It might also contribute to weight gain. Aim to get at least 6-7 hours of quality sleep each night.

Not Eating Enough Fruits and Vegetables

As you age, your calorie needs will also most likely reduce. However, you still need to consume enough fresh fruits and vegetables to ensure that you get that glow linked to healthy and graceful aging. Not including enough fruits and veggies in your diet might cause your complexion to age fast. You will develop more wrinkles. I highly advise putting more colorful fruits and veggies on your plate. Also, make sure that you stick to a diet composed of foods containing the heart-healthy Omega 3 and fiber.

Eating Too Much Sweets

Consuming sugary food excessively, whether it is soda, sugary cereals, or sugary nutrition bars, can also drain your fountain of youth. Foods that have extremely high sugar content have the tendency of overwhelming your body with sugar molecules. Such excessive amounts of sugar molecules can trigger vital proteins, such as elastin and collagen (yes, the ones designed to keep your skin look young and firm), to lessen their production.

It can also cause inflammation that might only lead to the acceleration of the aging process. Fortunately, you can reverse this by cutting out processed, fried, and sugary foods from your diet.

Not Doing Enough Physical Activities

Even in your 50s, you still need to incorporate a physical activity or two in your daily routines. In fact, moderate walking for just 30 minutes every day is already enough to improve your health, strengthen your bones, improve your insulin sensitivity, protect your heart, and reduce the bad cholesterol present in your body. With proper exercise and activity, you can lower your chance of gaining too much weight. You can stay fit and fab even as you age.

Chapter 9 – How to Stay on Track?

During my journey to maintaining a healthy weight, one thing I noticed is that the hardest part linked to it, is actually staying on track. With too many temptations around, I had a difficult time staying committed to my target weight, after I lose the initial few pounds. Some of those who successfully shed weight and achieved their dream figure at that age may have a difficult time staying on track.

Fortunately, there are some things you can do to ensure that you stay committed to your journey to maintaining a healthy weight and aging gracefully.

#1 – Weigh Yourself Regularly

Make it a point to keep track of your weight. Step on the scale regularly as that's a very helpful tool in maintaining your weight. It lets you become more aware of your progress while encouraging good weight control behaviors. I also noticed that weighing myself regularly caused me to eat fewer calories all throughout the day, causing me to stick to my target weight.

In your case, the number of times you weigh yourself is actually based on your personal preference and what works for you. You may choose to weigh yourself daily or do it once or twice every week.

#2 – Monitor your Carb Intake

Staying on track of your weight loss goals is easier to achieve if you pay close attention to your carb intake, particularly the specific amount and type you take in. Even if you've already reached your target weight, you still need to stick to healthy eating. Avoid eating excessive amounts of refined carbs, like those found in fruit juices, white pasta, and white bread, as these can negatively affect your goal to maintain your weight.

You need to limit your overall carb consumption so you can keep a close watch on your weight. Note that sticking to a low-carb diet after losing weight will let you maintain your new weight for a long time. Sticking to a low-carb diet can also lessen your risk of consuming more calories than the amount you burn.

#3 – Avoid Criticizing Yourself Too Much

If you want to stay on track for your fitness, then make it a point to set realistic goals. Being realistic in your journey towards maintaining your fit body will prevent you from dealing with disappointments in the long run. You should also avoid berating yourself too much for all the shortcomings and failures that you will encounter during your journey. Note that excessive self-criticism will only cause you to lose your confidence and increase the level of your anxiety.

This will also trigger stress, causing your body to respond through adrenaline and cortisol. Such natural reaction will lower your immunity, cause exhaustion and weariness, and slow down your metabolism. Worse, it can trigger emotional eating or cravings for unhealthy stuff. If that happens, then you are only pushing yourself to gain weight once again.

If you want to continue your success in maintaining your weight, then give yourself a positive reassurance instead of unnecessary criticisms. Put your mind at ease by reminding yourself that you're capable of maintaining your fabulous look and figure after 50.

Conclusion – New Me; New Life

Healthy eating and proper exercise are definitely among the best ways for you to stay healthy and sexy even after you reach 50. I realized how helpful both these habits are in maintaining my figure. I'm sure that sticking to a healthy diet and performing regular exercises can also help those who wish to age gracefully.

Now that you're aware of how to lose weight over 50, it's time to apply what you've learned. Embrace the new you and your new life as you embark on a new chapter of your life. Rest assured that all the tips and routines I included in this book are designed to guide you in making the transition much easier to handle. The guide can even help you handle some of the unwanted menopausal symptoms.

Apart from the provided tips, I also highly recommend accepting and embracing your own body. Appreciating your body can further motivate you to take good care of yourself. This will result in better nutritional and fitness habits, allowing you to lose weight, maintain your figure, and enjoy graceful aging.

-- Erika Bates

www.ingramcontent.com/pod-product-compliance
Lightning Source LLC
Chambersburg PA
CBHW070233260726
48658CB00006BA/2308